From Classroom to Clinic: Medicinal Botany

for Student Practitioners

Mark Twain

From Classroom to Clinic: Medicinal Botany for Student Practitioners

Copyright © 2023 by Mark Twain

The first edition was published in 2023

ISBN:
Published by:
Sunshine
1663 Liberty Drive
Hyderabad, IN 47403
www.Sunshinepublishers.com

This book is self-published using on-demand printing and publishing, which allows it to be printed and distributed globally

TABLE OF CONTENT

Chapter 10: Conclusion and Practical Applications

Recapitulation of Key Concepts

Recommendations for Student Practitioners

Prospect for Further Research in Medicinal Botany

Chapter 1: Introduction to Medicinal Botany

The Importance of Medicinal Botany in Healthcare

Introduction:

In the world of healthcare, the use of medicinal plants has been a longstanding tradition that dates back centuries. Today, as we delve into the fascinating realm of medicinal botany, we will explore the vital role this field plays in our modern healthcare system. As students with a keen interest in botany, it is crucial to understand how the study of medicinal plants can contribute to our future roles as healthcare practitioners.

Exploring Nature's Pharmacy:

Medicinal botany opens the doors to nature's vast pharmacy, offering a wide range of plants with therapeutic properties. Through careful research and analysis, scientists have discovered numerous bioactive compounds present in plants that can be harnessed for medicinal purposes. These compounds, such as alkaloids, flavonoids, and terpenes, have the potential to treat various diseases and conditions.

Understanding the Connection:

As students of botany, it is essential to comprehend the intimate relationship between plants and humans. Medicinal botany helps us understand how plants have adapted to produce these bioactive compounds as a means of defense against pests and pathogens. By studying the chemical composition and biological activity of these compounds, we can unlock their potential for human health and well-being.

Contributions to Healthcare:

Medicinal botany plays a significant role in healthcare by providing a vast array of natural remedies and alternative treatments. Many well-established pharmaceutical drugs, such as aspirin and morphine, originated from plant sources. Furthermore, medicinal plants are often used in traditional medicine practices across the globe, where they have been trusted for generations.

Enhancing Drug Discovery:

In addition to the traditional uses of medicinal plants, the field of medicinal botany is also crucial in drug discovery and development. By studying the chemical composition and biological activity of various plants, scientists can identify potential leads for new pharmaceutical drugs. This process, known as pharmacognosy, allows researchers to harness the power of nature to address unmet medical needs.

Conservation and Sustainability:

As students of botany, we must also recognize the importance of conservation and sustainability in medicinal botany. With the increasing demand for medicinal plants, it is crucial to ensure their long-term availability. By studying plant habitats, ecology, and cultivation techniques, we can contribute to the sustainable use and conservation of these valuable resources.

Conclusion:

In conclusion, the study of medicinal botany is of utmost importance for students interested in botany and healthcare. By understanding the intricate relationship between plants and humans, we can harness the healing properties of nature's pharmacy. Through contributions to healthcare, drug discovery, and conservation efforts, medicinal botany has the potential to revolutionize the way we approach healthcare. As future practitioners, let us embrace the vast potential of medicinal botany and work towards a healthier future for all.

The Role of Medicinal Botany in Student Practice

In the field of botany, the study of medicinal plants holds a significant place. The exploration of the therapeutic properties of plants has been a subject of fascination for centuries. From ancient civilizations to modern times, medicinal botany has played a crucial role in the development of medicine. For students pursuing a career in botany, understanding the role of medicinal plants in their practice is essential.

Medicinal botany involves the study of plants and their active compounds that have medicinal properties. These plants have been used for centuries to treat various ailments and are an integral part of traditional medicine systems around the world. By delving into this field, students gain a deep understanding of the intricate relationship between plants and human health.

One of the key benefits of studying medicinal botany is the opportunity to discover new sources of medicine. With the increasing prevalence of drug-resistant pathogens and the side effects associated with synthetic drugs, the search for natural remedies has become more crucial than ever. Students can contribute to this search by identifying and studying plants that possess medicinal potential. Their research and findings may help in the development of new drugs or alternative treatments.

Furthermore, studying medicinal botany equips students with invaluable knowledge about plant identification and taxonomy. Identifying plants accurately is vital, as different species may have different therapeutic properties. By learning about plant morphology, taxonomy, and identification techniques, students can confidently identify and utilize medicinal plants in their practice.

Additionally, medicinal botany provides students with a holistic approach to healthcare. By understanding the medicinal properties of plants, students can explore natural therapies that may complement conventional treatments. This integrative approach can offer patients a wider range of treatment options and potentially reduce reliance on synthetic drugs.

Moreover, exploring medicinal botany enhances students' understanding of the importance of biodiversity conservation. Many medicinal plants are endangered or at risk due to deforestation, habitat destruction, and unsustainable harvesting. By studying medicinal botany, students become advocates for the preservation and sustainable use of these plant species, contributing to the conservation of natural resources.

In conclusion, the role of medicinal botany in student practice is crucial for aspiring botanists. By studying medicinal plants, students can contribute to the development of new medicines, gain expertise in plant identification, embrace a holistic approach to healthcare, and actively participate in biodiversity conservation. Understanding the therapeutic properties of plants opens up a world of possibilities for students in the field of botany, making it an indispensable area of study for those passionate about both plants and human health.

Chapter 2: Fundamentals of Botany

Plant Anatomy and Physiology

In the vast world of botany, understanding plant anatomy and physiology is paramount for any aspiring student practitioner. This subchapter will delve into the intricate details of how plants function and how their structures contribute to their overall health and medicinal properties.

Plant anatomy refers to the study of the internal structures of plants. By examining the various tissues, cells, and organs that make up a plant, we can gain insight into their growth, development, and overall function. Students of botany must familiarize themselves with the different types of tissues such as dermal, ground, and vascular, and how they work together to support plant growth and survival.

Additionally, understanding plant physiology is crucial for comprehending the processes that occur within plants to maintain their health and vitality. From photosynthesis to respiration, plants rely on a complex network of biochemical reactions to produce energy and essential compounds. By delving into the intricacies of these processes, students can gain insights into the therapeutic properties of medicinal plants.

Furthermore, this subchapter will explore the relationship between plant anatomy and physiology and the production of secondary metabolites. These compounds, often responsible for a plant's medicinal properties, are synthesized within specific plant tissues and play a vital role in defense mechanisms and interactions with their environment. By understanding the anatomy and physiology of a plant, students can identify the specific tissues and organs responsible for the production of these valuable compounds.

Moreover, this subchapter will cover the role of environmental factors such as light, temperature, and water availability on plant anatomy and physiology. By understanding how plants respond to their surroundings, students can optimize growth conditions for medicinal plants and enhance their therapeutic potential.

Throughout this subchapter, practical examples and case studies will be provided to bridge the gap between classroom knowledge and real-world application. Students will gain a deeper understanding of how plant anatomy and physiology directly impact the efficacy of herbal remedies and the development of pharmaceutical drugs.

In summary, "Plant Anatomy and Physiology" is a pivotal subchapter in the book "From Classroom to Clinic: Medicinal Botany for Student Practitioners." It provides students with a comprehensive understanding of how plants function at the anatomical and physiological level, emphasizing the relevance of these concepts in the field of botany. By exploring the intricate details of plant structures and their functions, students will be equipped with the knowledge necessary to identify, cultivate, and utilize medicinal plants for the betterment of human health.

Classification and Taxonomy of Medicinal Plants

Understanding the classification and taxonomy of medicinal plants is essential for students pursuing a career in botany. This subchapter aims to provide a comprehensive overview of the principles and methods used for categorizing and organizing medicinal plants based on their characteristics and properties.

Classification is the process of grouping organisms into categories based on their shared characteristics. Taxonomy, on the other hand, is the science of naming, describing, and classifying organisms. In the realm of medicinal plants, classification and taxonomy play a crucial role in identifying, studying, and utilizing these valuable resources.

The classification of medicinal plants is typically based on various factors, including their morphological features, chemical composition, and therapeutic properties. By examining the overall structure, shape, and size of the plant, botanists can determine its taxonomic family, genus, and species. This information is then used to create a standardized naming system, ensuring that each plant is uniquely identified.

Taxonomy provides a systematic approach to organizing medicinal plants, enabling researchers and practitioners to easily access information about their properties, uses, and potential therapeutic benefits. The classification system allows for the comparison and analysis of plants within the same family or genus, aiding in the discovery of new medicinal compounds and the development of targeted treatments.

During the classification process, medicinal plants are often grouped based on their therapeutic properties and the ailments they can address. For example, plants with antimicrobial properties may be categorized separately from those used to treat digestive disorders or respiratory conditions. This organization allows students to easily navigate the vast world of medicinal plants, enabling them to understand and appreciate the diversity and potential of these natural remedies.

Furthermore, studying the classification and taxonomy of medicinal plants allows students to explore the evolutionary relationships between different species. By examining the similarities and differences in their genetic makeup, students can gain insights into the evolutionary history and origins of these plants. This knowledge is invaluable when it comes to understanding their adaptability, distribution, and potential for cultivation.

In conclusion, the classification and taxonomy of medicinal plants are fundamental aspects of the study of botany. By categorizing and organizing these plants based on their characteristics and properties, students can navigate the vast world of medicinal plants with ease. This knowledge not only aids in identification and understanding but also opens doors to the discovery of new medicinal compounds and the development of targeted treatments.

Plant Growth and Development

In the fascinating world of botany, understanding plant growth and development is crucial for student practitioners looking to delve into the realms of medicinal plants. This subchapter aims to provide a comprehensive overview of the processes involved in the growth and development of plants, offering valuable insights for students in the field of botany.

Plant growth encompasses the increase in size and mass of plants over time. It is driven by two main factors: cell division and cell expansion. Cell division allows plants to increase their cell numbers, leading to overall growth, while cell expansion enables the enlargement of individual cells. These processes, influenced by various internal and external factors, contribute to the overall development of plants.

External factors such as light, temperature, water availability, and nutrient supply play vital roles in plant growth and development. Through photosynthesis, plants utilize sunlight to convert carbon dioxide and water into sugars, which fuel their growth. Understanding the interplay between light and plant growth is of utmost importance to student practitioners, as it directly affects the production of medicinal compounds within plants.

Additionally, hormones play a pivotal role in plant growth and development. Phytohormones, also known as plant hormones, regulate various processes such as cell division, elongation, and differentiation. Auxins, for example, control cell elongation and are involved in tropisms, which are plant movements in response to external stimuli. Gibberellins, on the other hand, stimulate cell division and elongation, promoting overall plant growth.

Plant development refers to the progression of plants from germination to maturity. It involves various stages, including seed germination, vegetative growth, and reproductive development. Student practitioners must understand these stages, as they impact the medicinal properties of plants. For instance, the concentration of active compounds may vary during different stages of plant development, influencing the potency and effectiveness of medicinal plant extracts.

By comprehending the intricacies of plant growth and development, student practitioners can optimize their cultivation and harvesting techniques to obtain plants with desired medicinal properties. Moreover, a deeper understanding of these processes enables the identification and extraction of potent medicinal compounds from plants, providing valuable resources for future clinical applications.

In conclusion, this subchapter on plant growth and development provides student practitioners in the field of botany with a comprehensive understanding of the processes that drive the growth and development of plants. By exploring the interplay between external factors, hormones, and plant development stages, students can harness this knowledge to cultivate and harvest medicinal plants with enhanced therapeutic potential.

Chapter 3: Principles of Medicinal Botany

Active Chemical Components in Medicinal Plants

In the field of medicinal botany, understanding the active chemical components present in plants is crucial for harnessing their therapeutic potential. Medicinal plants have been used for centuries in traditional medicine systems worldwide, and their active chemical compounds have played a significant role in treating various ailments. This subchapter aims to provide students with an overview of the active chemical components found in medicinal plants and their importance in healthcare.

One of the primary classes of active chemical components in medicinal plants are alkaloids. Alkaloids are organic compounds that often contain nitrogen and exhibit diverse physiological effects. Examples include morphine from the opium poppy (Papaver somniferum), which acts as a potent pain reliever, and caffeine from coffee (Coffea spp.), which stimulates the central nervous system. Understanding the alkaloids present in medicinal plants is essential for identifying their therapeutic benefits and potential side effects.

Another significant class of active chemical components are terpenoids. Terpenoids are a diverse group of compounds that are responsible for the aroma and flavor of many plants. They have been widely studied for their medicinal properties, including antimicrobial, anti-inflammatory, and anticancer activities. For instance, the essential oil of lavender (Lavandula angustifolia) contains terpenoids such as linalool, which possesses sedative and anxiolytic effects. Studying terpenoids in medicinal plants allows students to explore their potential applications in drug development and alternative therapies.

Phenolic compounds, such as flavonoids and tannins, are also important active chemical components in medicinal plants. These compounds possess antioxidant properties and have been associated with various health benefits, including cardiovascular protection and anticancer effects. For example, quercetin, a flavonoid found in many plants, has been shown to have anti-inflammatory and antiviral activities. Understanding the role of phenolic compounds in medicinal plants provides students with insights into their potential therapeutic applications and their beneficial effects on human health.

In conclusion, studying the active chemical components in medicinal plants is essential for student practitioners in the field of medicinal botany. Alkaloids, terpenoids, and phenolic compounds are just a few examples of the diverse range of active chemical components found in these plants. By understanding their properties and potential therapeutic applications, students can unlock the immense potential of medicinal plants in healthcare.

Extraction and Isolation Techniques

In the world of medicinal botany, the extraction and isolation of active compounds from plants are essential steps towards developing effective medicines. This subchapter explores the various techniques used in extracting and isolating these compounds, providing students with a comprehensive understanding of the process.

1.   Introduction   to   Extraction   Techniques: The subchapter begins with an introduction to extraction techniques, highlighting their importance in isolating active compounds from plants. Students will learn about the different extraction methods, such as maceration, percolation, and distillation, and how each technique is suitable for specific plant materials.

2.   Solvent   Selection   and   Solvent-Solute   Interaction: Understanding the properties of solvents and their interaction with solutes is crucial for successful extraction. This section delves into the selection of appropriate solvents based on their polarity and extraction efficiency. Students will also learn about the factors that influence solvent-solute interaction, such as temperature, pH, and time.

3.   Common   Extraction   Techniques: This section provides an in-depth exploration of common extraction techniques used in medicinal botany. Students will learn about techniques like Soxhlet extraction, liquid-liquid extraction, and supercritical fluid extraction, along with their advantages and limitations. Case studies and practical examples will be included to facilitate a better understanding.

4. Isolation Techniques:
Once the active compounds are extracted, the next step is their isolation. This section focuses on various isolation techniques employed in medicinal botany, such as chromatography (thin-layer chromatography, column chromatography) and crystallization. Students will gain insights into the principles behind these techniques and their application in the separation of complex mixtures.

5. Analytical Techniques for Compound Identification:
After isolation, compound identification becomes crucial. Students will be introduced to various analytical techniques like spectrophotometry, nuclear magnetic resonance (NMR), and mass spectrometry (MS). The subchapter will explain how these techniques help in determining the structure, purity, and quantity of isolated compounds.

6. Ethical Considerations and Sustainability:
In the final section, ethical considerations and sustainability aspects related to extraction and isolation techniques will be discussed. Students will learn about environmentally friendly extraction methods, the importance of plant conservation, and the ethical sourcing of plant materials.

This subchapter on extraction and isolation techniques provides students with a comprehensive understanding of the processes involved in medicinal botany. By exploring various techniques, solvents, and analytical methods, students will gain the knowledge and skills necessary to contribute to the development of effective medicines while upholding ethical and sustainable practices within the field of botany.

Pharmacological Properties of Medicinal Plants

In the vast realm of medicinal botany, understanding the pharmacological properties of plants is of utmost importance for aspiring student practitioners. This subchapter delves into the fascinating world of pharmacological properties of medicinal plants, providing students with a comprehensive overview of how certain plants can be harnessed for their therapeutic benefits.

Pharmacological properties refer to the physiological effects that medicinal plants have on the human body. These properties determine the potential uses and applications of plants in treating various ailments and diseases. By exploring the pharmacological properties of medicinal plants, students can gain a deeper understanding of how these plants interact with the human body, paving the way for effective herbal remedies.

One key aspect covered in this subchapter is the identification and extraction of active compounds from medicinal plants. Students will learn about the different classes of compounds, such as alkaloids, flavonoids, terpenoids, and phenolic compounds, that contribute to the medicinal properties of plants. Understanding the chemical composition of plants is crucial in determining their potential pharmacological activities.

The subchapter also focuses on the diverse range of pharmacological properties exhibited by medicinal plants. Students will explore plants with analgesic properties, which can alleviate pain, and plants with anti-inflammatory properties, which can reduce inflammation in the body. Additionally, they will learn about plants with antimicrobial properties, which can combat bacterial, fungal, and viral infections, and plants with antioxidant properties, which can protect against oxidative stress and cellular damage.

Furthermore, this subchapter delves into the importance of conducting pharmacological studies and clinical trials to validate the efficacy and safety of medicinal plants. Students will gain insights into the methodologies used in these studies, including in vitro and in vivo experiments, as well as the ethical considerations involved.

To enhance the learning experience, case studies of specific medicinal plants will be presented, highlighting their pharmacological properties and therapeutic applications. Students will be encouraged to critically analyze these case studies, fostering a deeper understanding of the complexities and potential limitations of using medicinal plants in clinical practice.

Overall, this subchapter on the pharmacological properties of medicinal plants provides botany students with a solid foundation in understanding the therapeutic potential of plants. By equipping them with this knowledge, it empowers future practitioners to explore and harness the immense healing power of nature in their clinical endeavors.

Chapter 4: Medicinal Plants Used in Traditional Medicine

Traditional Medicinal Systems and their Importance

In the world of medicinal botany, it is essential for students to understand the significance of traditional medicinal systems. These systems, which have been practiced by various cultures for centuries, offer a wealth of knowledge and remedies that can greatly benefit modern medicine. This subchapter aims to delve into the importance of traditional medicinal systems and highlight their relevance to students in the field of botany.

Traditional medicinal systems, such as Ayurveda, Traditional Chinese Medicine (TCM), and Indigenous healing practices, have deep roots in the use of plants for therapeutic purposes. These systems recognize the intricate relationship between human beings and nature, emphasizing the need for balance and harmony within the body. By understanding traditional medicinal systems, students can gain valuable insights into the historical and cultural context of botanical medicine.

One of the key reasons traditional medicinal systems are important is their extensive knowledge of plant properties and their therapeutic uses. Throughout history, indigenous communities and ancient civilizations have accumulated a vast body of knowledge regarding the medicinal properties of plants. This knowledge has been passed down through generations, serving as the foundation for many modern pharmaceuticals and treatments. By studying traditional medicinal systems, students can tap into this wisdom, discovering new plant-based remedies and expanding their understanding of plant chemistry.

Furthermore, traditional medicinal systems often take a holistic approach to healthcare, focusing not only on the physical symptoms but also on the mental, emotional, and spiritual well-being of individuals. This comprehensive approach recognizes the interconnectedness of various body systems and the importance of addressing the root causes of illnesses. Students can learn from these systems and incorporate holistic perspectives into their future practice, providing well-rounded care to their patients.

Moreover, traditional medicinal systems highlight the importance of sustainability and conservation of plant resources. Many of these systems have developed methods for ethically harvesting and cultivating medicinal plants, ensuring their availability for future generations. With the current environmental challenges, it is essential for botany students to embrace sustainable practices and contribute to the preservation of plant biodiversity.

In conclusion, traditional medicinal systems offer a wealth of knowledge and practices that can greatly enhance the field of botanical medicine. By studying these systems, students can expand their understanding of plant properties, embrace holistic approaches to healthcare, and contribute to the sustainability of medicinal plants. This subchapter serves as a gateway to exploring the importance and relevance of traditional medicinal systems for students in the field of botany.

Common Medicinal Plants in Traditional Medicine

In the field of botany, the study of medicinal plants holds significant importance. Traditional medicine, also known as herbal medicine, has been practiced for centuries across various cultures. It involves the use of plants and plant extracts to treat and prevent diseases. In this subchapter, we will explore some common medicinal plants used in traditional medicine, providing students with valuable insights into the world of botanical medicine.

One of the most widely recognized medicinal plants is Aloe vera. This succulent plant has a gel-like substance in its leaves, which is known for its healing properties. Aloe vera is used topically to soothe burns, wounds, and skin irritations. It also has antimicrobial and anti-inflammatory properties, making it a versatile herb in traditional medicine.

Another prominent medicinal plant is Echinacea, commonly known as purple coneflower. Echinacea is native to North America and has been used by Native American tribes for centuries to boost the immune system and treat infections. It is believed to have antiviral and antibacterial properties and is often used to prevent and treat the common cold and flu.

Ginger, a popular spice, is also a well-known medicinal plant. It has a long history of use in traditional medicine for its digestive properties. Ginger is often used to relieve nausea, vomiting, and indigestion. It also has anti-inflammatory effects and can help alleviate pain associated with arthritis.

Turmeric, a bright yellow spice commonly used in Indian cuisine, is another powerful medicinal plant. Curcumin, the active compound in turmeric, has potent antioxidant and anti-inflammatory properties. It is believed to have numerous health benefits, including reducing the risk of chronic diseases such as heart disease, cancer, and Alzheimer's.

Lastly, we cannot overlook the medicinal properties of garlic. Garlic has been used for its medicinal properties for thousands of years. It contains sulfur compounds that have antimicrobial and immune-boosting properties. Garlic is often used to lower blood pressure, reduce cholesterol levels, and boost the immune system.

As aspiring botany students, understanding the role of these common medicinal plants in traditional medicine is crucial. By delving into the world of herbal medicine, students can gain a deeper appreciation for the potential benefits that plants offer in promoting health and preventing diseases. Furthermore, this knowledge can be applied in clinical settings, where patients may seek alternative or complementary treatments.

In conclusion, the study of common medicinal plants in traditional medicine is an essential aspect of botany. Through exploring plants like Aloe vera, Echinacea, ginger, turmeric, and garlic, students can broaden their understanding of the medicinal properties and potential applications of these botanical treasures. By embracing the knowledge of traditional medicine, future practitioners can bridge the gap between the classroom and the clinic, offering a comprehensive approach to patient care.

Ethnobotanical Research and Documentation

In the field of botany, one of the most fascinating and multidisciplinary areas of study is ethnobotany. This subchapter will delve into the world of ethnobotanical research and documentation, shedding light on the importance of this field for student practitioners in botany.

Ethnobotany is the scientific study of the relationships between people and plants. It encompasses various disciplines such as anthropology, ecology, and pharmacology, making it an incredibly diverse and exciting field to explore. By understanding the traditional knowledge, practices, and beliefs surrounding plants in different cultures, ethnobotanists can uncover valuable information about the potential medicinal properties of various plant species.

Ethnobotanical research involves conducting fieldwork, often in remote and culturally diverse areas, to document the traditional uses of plants by indigenous communities. This research not only helps preserve the knowledge of these communities but also provides valuable insights into the potential medicinal applications of plants. Through interviews, observations, and participatory approaches, student practitioners can contribute to the documentation of ethnomedicinal practices.

The documentation of ethnobotanical knowledge is crucial for several reasons. Firstly, it helps conserve traditional knowledge that has been passed down through generations. As cultures evolve and modernize, traditional practices can be lost, along with the valuable knowledge they contain. By documenting these practices, student practitioners can ensure their preservation for future generations.

Secondly, ethnobotanical research contributes to the development of new medicines. Many modern drugs have their origins in traditional plant-based remedies. By studying the traditional uses of plants, student practitioners can identify potential sources for new drugs and contribute to the development of alternative therapies.

Lastly, ethnobotanical research promotes cultural understanding and respect. By engaging with indigenous communities and valuing their traditional knowledge, student practitioners can foster positive relationships and promote cultural diversity.

In conclusion, ethnobotanical research and documentation play a vital role in the field of botany, offering a unique perspective on the relationship between people and plants. Student practitioners in botany have the opportunity to contribute to this field by conducting fieldwork, documenting traditional knowledge, and uncovering potential medicinal applications of plants. By preserving traditional practices, contributing to drug development, and promoting cultural understanding, student practitioners can help bridge the gap between classroom knowledge and real-world applications in the clinic.

Chapter 5: Medicinal Plants and Modern Medicine

Integration of Medicinal Plants into Modern Healthcare

In recent years, there has been a growing interest in the use of medicinal plants as a complementary approach to modern healthcare. This integration of traditional herbal remedies with modern medicine offers a promising avenue for students studying botany to explore. As future practitioners, it is crucial to understand the potential benefits and challenges associated with incorporating medicinal plants into contemporary healthcare practices.

The use of medicinal plants dates back thousands of years. Indigenous cultures across the globe have relied on the healing properties of various plants to treat ailments and maintain overall well-being. These traditional remedies often contain a rich array of bioactive compounds that can have significant therapeutic effects. As students of botany, it is essential to delve into the chemical composition of medicinal plants and understand how these compounds interact with the human body.

One of the key advantages of integrating medicinal plants into modern healthcare is the potential for natural remedies to complement conventional treatments. While pharmaceutical drugs have undoubtedly revolutionized healthcare, they often come with side effects and limitations. Medicinal plants, on the other hand, offer a more holistic approach, harnessing the synergistic effects of multiple compounds to address the root cause of diseases. This integration can also pave the way for personalized medicine, as the diverse array of plant species allows for tailored treatment options.

However, the integration of medicinal plants into modern healthcare is not without challenges. Standardization and quality control are vital aspects to consider. The potency and efficacy of herbal remedies can vary significantly depending on factors such as plant species, growing conditions, and preparation methods. As students, it is crucial to familiarize ourselves with proper cultivation techniques, extraction methods, and quality assurance protocols to ensure the safety and efficacy of medicinal plant-based treatments.

Furthermore, the ethical and sustainable use of medicinal plants is a critical consideration. As botany students, it is our responsibility to promote conservation efforts, preserve biodiversity, and support sustainable harvesting practices to prevent overexploitation and protect these valuable resources for future generations.

In conclusion, the integration of medicinal plants into modern healthcare presents an exciting opportunity for botany students. By understanding the chemical composition, therapeutic potential, and challenges associated with herbal remedies, we can contribute to the development of evidence-based, safe, and effective plant-based treatments. Through our knowledge and dedication, we can bridge the gap between traditional herbal medicine and modern healthcare, ultimately benefiting patients and advancing the field of botany.

Drug Discovery and Development from Medicinal Plants

In the field of botany, one of the fascinating areas of research is drug discovery and development from medicinal plants. This subchapter aims to introduce students to the exciting world of using plants as a source of potential therapeutic agents. By delving into this topic, students will gain a deeper understanding of the significance of plants in modern medicine.

Medicinal plants have been used for centuries by various cultures around the world to treat illnesses and ailments. These plants possess a vast array of chemical compounds that have the potential to be developed into drugs. The process of discovering and developing drugs from medicinal plants involves a multidisciplinary approach that combines botany, chemistry, pharmacology, and clinical research.

The subchapter will provide students with an overview of the different methods used in drug discovery and development. It will address the importance of plant collection, identification, and characterization, highlighting the significance of botanical gardens and herbaria in preserving and studying medicinal plants. Students will also learn about the extraction and isolation of bioactive compounds from plant materials, followed by various techniques used to evaluate their pharmacological activities.

Moreover, this subchapter will shed light on the challenges faced in drug discovery and development from medicinal plants. Students will understand the complexity of identifying and isolating active compounds from plant extracts, as well as the need for rigorous testing to ensure safety and efficacy. The importance of sustainable practices and conservation efforts will also be emphasized, as overexploitation of medicinal plants can lead to ecological imbalances.

To provide students with real-world examples, this subchapter will showcase some successful drugs derived from medicinal plants. These examples will demonstrate the immense potential of botanical resources in addressing various diseases, ranging from cancer and cardiovascular disorders to infectious diseases and neurodegenerative conditions. Students will gain insight into the rigorous process of clinical trials and regulatory approvals that a drug must undergo before reaching the market.

By the end of this subchapter, students will have a comprehensive understanding of the role of medicinal plants in drug discovery and development. They will appreciate the importance of preserving botanical diversity and the need for continued research in this promising field. Armed with this knowledge, students can contribute to the advancement of medicinal botany and make a positive impact on healthcare practices in the future.

Clinical Trials and Evidence-based Medicine

In the field of medicine, it is crucial for practitioners to rely on evidence-based practices to ensure the safety and effectiveness of treatments. Clinical trials play a vital role in this process, providing scientific evidence to support the use of medicinal botanicals. This subchapter will delve into the significance of clinical trials and evidence-based medicine in the realm of botany, equipping students with the essential knowledge to become proficient in their future roles as practitioners.

Clinical trials are rigorous scientific studies that evaluate the safety and efficacy of medicinal botanicals. These trials involve human participants who are carefully selected and closely monitored throughout the study. By following strict protocols, clinical trials aim to provide unbiased and reliable evidence on the benefits and risks associated with the use of specific plant-based treatments.

For students in the field of botany, understanding the importance of clinical trials is paramount. It allows them to critically evaluate the therapeutic claims made about medicinal plants and discern between evidence-based information and anecdotal knowledge. By analyzing the results of clinical trials, students can identify which plant-based medicines have been proven effective and safe for specific conditions.

Moreover, evidence-based medicine relies on the integration of clinical trial findings with the practitioner's expertise and patient values. As future practitioners, students need to be well-versed in evaluating the quality of clinical trials and assessing the relevance of their findings to individual patients. This skill is essential to provide personalized and effective botanical treatments.

Within this subchapter, students will be introduced to the different phases of clinical trials, from preclinical research to post-marketing surveillance. They will learn about the criteria for selecting participants, the importance of randomization and blinding, and the statistical analysis used in clinical trials. Additionally, students will explore the ethical considerations involved in conducting clinical trials, including informed consent and patient privacy.

By grasping the fundamentals of clinical trials and evidence-based medicine, students can navigate the complex world of medicinal botany with confidence. They will develop the skills necessary to critically evaluate scientific evidence, make informed decisions about treatment options, and ensure the well-being of their future patients.

Chapter 6: Cultivation and Conservation of Medicinal Plants

Sustainable Cultivation Practices

In the ever-growing field of medicinal botany, it is crucial for student practitioners to understand and implement sustainable cultivation practices. As future professionals in the field, it is our responsibility to ensure the long-term viability of medicinal plants for both ecological and human health purposes.

Sustainable cultivation practices promote the growth and preservation of medicinal plants while minimizing negative impacts on the environment. These practices enable us to meet the increasing demand for medicinal plants while also conserving biodiversity and protecting natural habitats. By adopting sustainable cultivation methods, we can contribute to the sustainability of the botanical medicine industry.

One key aspect of sustainable cultivation is the use of organic and natural farming techniques. This involves avoiding the use of synthetic pesticides, herbicides, and fertilizers that can harm both the plants and the environment. Instead, we can focus on utilizing natural alternatives such as compost, crop rotation, and biological pest control methods. By doing so, we can maintain the health and vitality of our medicinal plants while minimizing the release of harmful chemicals into the environment.

Another important practice is the conservation of water resources. Water is essential for the growth of medicinal plants, but it is also a limited resource. By implementing water-saving techniques such as drip irrigation, mulching, and rainwater harvesting, we can reduce water consumption while ensuring adequate hydration for our plants. This not only benefits the environment but also helps us become more efficient and responsible cultivators.

Furthermore, sustainable cultivation practices involve promoting biodiversity and protecting natural habitats. By growing medicinal plants in a way that mimics their natural environment, we can enhance their medicinal properties and preserve their genetic diversity. This can be achieved by creating small-scale ecosystems, incorporating companion planting, and avoiding the use of monocultures. By supporting biodiversity, we create a more resilient and sustainable environment for both plants and wildlife.

As students of botany, it is essential to understand and implement sustainable cultivation practices in our future careers as medicinal plant practitioners. By adopting these practices, we contribute to the conservation of our natural resources, protect the environment, and ensure the availability of medicinal plants for generations to come. Let us strive to be responsible stewards and advocates for sustainable cultivation, promoting a harmonious relationship between humans, plants, and the environment.

Plant Propagation Methods

Introduction:

Plant propagation is the process of creating new plants from existing ones, allowing botanists and horticulturists to cultivate and expand plant populations. This subchapter will provide an overview of various plant propagation methods used in the field of botany. Understanding these techniques is crucial for students studying medicinal botany as it enables them to reproduce and maintain specific plant species for research and clinical purposes.

1.   Sexual   Propagation:
Sexual propagation involves the union of male and female gametes, resulting in the formation of seeds. This method allows for genetic variation and is commonly used for plant breeding. Students will learn about pollination, fertilization, and seed development, as well as techniques for germinating seeds and caring for seedlings.

2.   Asexual   Propagation:
Asexual propagation, also known as vegetative propagation, does not involve the fusion of gametes and produces offspring that are genetically identical to the parent plant. This method is particularly useful for preserving desirable traits in plants. Students will explore techniques such as cutting, layering, grafting, and tissue culture, which allow for the multiplication of plants without the need for seeds.

3.   Cutting   Propagation:
Cutting propagation involves taking a piece of a plant, known as a cutting, and encouraging it to develop roots to form a new plant. This method is commonly used for woody plants such as shrubs and trees.

Students will learn about different types of cuttings, rooting hormones, and proper environmental conditions required for successful rooting.

4. Layering Propagation: Layering is a method in which a portion of a plant's stem is bent and covered with soil to encourage root development. This technique is particularly suitable for plants with flexible stems, such as vines and climbers. Students will explore various layering techniques, including simple layering, air layering, and tip layering.

5. Grafting Propagation: Grafting involves joining two different plant parts, known as the scion and the rootstock, to create a new plant with desirable traits. This method allows for the combination of different cultivars or species, resulting in plants with unique characteristics. Students will be introduced to the different types of grafting, such as whip and tongue grafting, cleft grafting, and bud grafting.

6. Tissue Culture: Tissue culture, also known as micropropagation, involves growing plant cells or tissues in a laboratory setting under sterile conditions. This technique allows for the rapid production of numerous identical plantlets, making it an essential tool in the propagation of rare or endangered plant species. Students will learn about the steps involved in tissue culture, including explant selection, sterilization, and nutrient media preparation.

Conclusion:

Understanding plant propagation methods is vital for students in the field of botany, especially those studying medicinal plants. By mastering these techniques, students can effectively cultivate and maintain plant populations for research, conservation, and clinical applications. Whether through sexual propagation, asexual propagation, or advanced techniques like tissue culture, students can contribute to the preservation and advancement of botanical knowledge for the benefit of future generations.

Conservation Strategies for Medicinal Plants

In the field of botany, the study and conservation of medicinal plants play a crucial role in preserving the world's biodiversity and the health of human populations. As aspiring botanists and student practitioners, it is essential for us to understand the importance of conservation strategies for medicinal plants and actively contribute to their preservation. This subchapter will delve into the various conservation strategies that can be implemented to protect and sustain these valuable plant species.

One of the primary strategies for conserving medicinal plants is the establishment and management of botanical gardens and arboretums. These institutions serve as living repositories of plant diversity, allowing for the cultivation and preservation of various medicinal plant species. Botanical gardens also provide an educational platform for students and the public to learn about the importance of medicinal plants, their traditional uses, and their potential in modern medicine.

Another crucial strategy is the protection and management of natural habitats where medicinal plants thrive. This involves identifying and assessing areas of high biodiversity, such as forests, wetlands, and grasslands, and implementing conservation measures to safeguard these habitats from destruction and degradation. Through the establishment of protected areas and the enforcement of strict regulations, we can ensure the long-term survival of medicinal plant populations.

In addition to habitat conservation, sustainable harvesting practices are vital for the survival of medicinal plants. Students must learn to identify and collect plant material responsibly, considering the plant's life cycle, population size, and regeneration capacity. Implementing sustainable harvesting practices includes techniques such as selective harvesting, which involves harvesting only a portion of the plant or only certain plant parts, allowing the remaining population to continue thriving.

Collaboration between botanists, local communities, and indigenous peoples is also crucial in the conservation of medicinal plants. By involving local knowledge and traditional practices, we can gain a deeper understanding of the ecological relationships and sustainable harvesting methods that have been employed for centuries. This collaborative approach fosters knowledge exchange, respect for cultural diversity, and ensures the equitable sharing of benefits derived from medicinal plant resources.

Lastly, research and development efforts should focus on the cultivation and propagation of endangered medicinal plant species. By studying their growth requirements, reproductive biology, and cultivation techniques, we can establish ex-situ conservation methods, such as seed banks and tissue culture, to safeguard these plants from extinction.

In conclusion, the conservation of medicinal plants is a pressing issue in the field of botany. As students and future practitioners, it is our responsibility to actively engage in the implementation of conservation strategies. By establishing botanical gardens, protecting natural habitats, promoting sustainable harvesting practices, fostering collaboration, and investing in research and development, we can contribute to the preservation of medicinal plant species for generations to come. Together, we can ensure that the invaluable knowledge and benefits derived from these plants are sustained and shared with the world.

Chapter 7: Safety and Quality Control in Medicinal Botany

Adverse Effects and Toxicity Screening

In the field of medicinal botany, it is essential for student practitioners to have a comprehensive understanding of the potential adverse effects and toxicity of medicinal plants. While plants have provided numerous therapeutic benefits to humans for centuries, it is important to recognize that they can also pose risks if used improperly or without the necessary precautions. This subchapter will delve into the various aspects of adverse effects and toxicity screening, equipping students with the knowledge needed to ensure safe and effective use of medicinal plants.

To begin, understanding adverse effects is crucial. Students will learn about the different types of adverse effects that can occur, including allergic reactions, gastrointestinal disturbances, and drug interactions. By exploring case studies and real-life examples, students will gain insights into the potential risks associated with specific medicinal plants. This knowledge will enable them to identify and manage adverse effects in their future practices.

Furthermore, the subchapter will cover the importance of toxicity screening. Students will explore the various methods used to evaluate the toxicity of medicinal plants, such as acute and chronic toxicity testing, genotoxicity testing, and reproductive toxicity screening. By familiarizing themselves with these screening methods, students will be able to assess the safety profile of a medicinal plant and make informed decisions regarding its use.

In addition, students will delve into the concept of dose-response relationships and therapeutic indices. This understanding will enable them to determine the appropriate dosage of a medicinal plant to achieve therapeutic effects while minimizing the risk of toxicity. They will also learn about factors that can influence toxicity, such as plant part used, preparation method, and individual variations in metabolism.

To enhance the learning experience, this subchapter will include interactive activities and case studies to allow students to apply their knowledge in real-world scenarios. They will have the opportunity to analyze toxicological data, interpret results, and make informed recommendations regarding the safe and effective use of medicinal plants.

By the end of this subchapter on adverse effects and toxicity screening, students will be equipped with the necessary knowledge and skills to navigate the potential risks associated with medicinal plants. They will be able to assess the safety profile of different plants, identify potential adverse effects, and make informed decisions in their future practices as botanical practitioners. This subchapter serves as a vital foundation for students pursuing a career in medicinal botany, ensuring that they prioritize patient safety while harnessing the therapeutic benefits of nature's pharmacy.

Good Manufacturing Practices for Herbal Products

In the world of herbal medicine, the quality and safety of herbal products are of utmost importance. As students of botany, it is essential for us to understand and adhere to Good Manufacturing Practices (GMP) when it comes to producing herbal products. This subchapter aims to provide an overview of GMP for herbal products, ensuring that our future endeavors in the field align with industry standards.

GMP for herbal products encompasses a set of guidelines and regulations that ensure the consistent quality, safety, and efficacy of herbal medicines. These practices cover various aspects of production, including cultivation, harvesting, processing, and packaging. By following GMP, we not only guarantee the quality of the final product but also promote consumer confidence in herbal medicine.

One crucial aspect of GMP is the cultivation and harvesting of medicinal plants. It is essential to select appropriate plant species, ensure proper soil conditions, and use organic cultivation methods. Adhering to sustainable harvesting practices helps preserve the natural resources and maintain the ecological balance. Additionally, proper post-harvest handling and storage techniques prevent the loss of active constituents in the plants.

Processing and manufacturing of herbal products must be done in a controlled environment to avoid contamination and maintain product integrity. GMP guidelines emphasize the use of standardized manufacturing processes, ensuring consistent quality and potency.

Regular equipment maintenance and calibration are vital to prevent cross-contamination and ensure accurate measurements.

Quality control plays a significant role in GMP for herbal products. It involves testing raw materials, intermediate products, and final products to ensure they meet predetermined quality standards. Various analytical techniques, such as high-performance liquid chromatography (HPLC), are employed to identify and quantify active constituents in herbal products. In addition, microbial and heavy metal testing is conducted to ensure product safety.

Packaging and labeling are also important aspects of GMP. Herbal products should be packaged in a way that preserves their quality and prevents contamination. Clear and accurate labeling ensures that consumers have all the necessary information about the product, including its ingredients, dosage, and contraindications.

By adhering to GMP for herbal products, we contribute to the overall quality and safety of herbal medicine. As future practitioners, it is our responsibility to produce and promote herbal products that meet the highest industry standards. Understanding and implementing GMP will not only enhance our credibility but also ensure the well-being of those who rely on herbal medicine for their health and wellness.

Quality Assurance and Standardization of Medicinal Botanicals

In the field of botanical medicine, quality assurance and standardization play a crucial role in ensuring the safety and efficacy of medicinal botanicals. As students of botany, it is essential to understand the importance of these processes and how they contribute to the development of effective herbal products.

Quality assurance refers to the systematic measures taken to ensure that medicinal botanicals meet predetermined standards of quality, purity, and safety. It involves various stages, starting from the selection of appropriate plant material to the final product's testing and evaluation. A robust quality assurance program helps prevent the presence of contaminants, adulterants, or undesirable substances in medicinal botanicals, thereby safeguarding the health of consumers.

Standardization, on the other hand, involves establishing uniformity in the composition and potency of medicinal botanicals. It ensures that each batch of a botanical product contains consistent amounts of active constituents, allowing for predictable therapeutic effects. Standardization typically involves the identification and quantification of marker compounds, which serve as indicators of the product's quality and potency. These markers are often specific to the plant species and are chosen based on their therapeutic relevance.

To achieve quality assurance and standardization, several techniques and methodologies are employed. These may include botanical identification using macroscopic and microscopic characteristics, chemical profiling using chromatographic techniques, and evaluation of active constituents through various analytical methods.

Additionally, good manufacturing practices (GMP) and quality control procedures are implemented to ensure compliance with regulatory standards and guidelines.

Students of botany should familiarize themselves with these techniques and methodologies, as they will be responsible for ensuring the quality and safety of medicinal botanicals in their future careers. By understanding and implementing quality assurance and standardization processes, they can contribute to the development of reliable herbal products and promote the integration of botanical medicine into mainstream healthcare.

It is important to note that quality assurance and standardization are ongoing processes that require continuous monitoring and improvement. As new scientific advancements and research emerge, it is necessary to update and adapt these processes to ensure the highest level of quality and safety in medicinal botanicals.

In conclusion, quality assurance and standardization are vital aspects of medicinal botany. Students of botany play a crucial role in ensuring the quality and safety of botanical products through their understanding and implementation of these processes. By upholding rigorous standards, they contribute to the development of effective herbal medicines that can be trusted by both healthcare practitioners and consumers.

Chapter 8: Case Studies in Medicinal Botany

Case Study 1: Medicinal Plant X for Disease Y

Introduction:

Welcome to the first case study in our book "From Classroom to Clinic: Medicinal Botany for Student Practitioners." In this chapter, we will delve into the fascinating world of medicinal plants and their potential in treating specific diseases. Our focus today is on Medicinal Plant X and its potential therapeutic benefits for Disease Y. This case study will serve as a practical example for students interested in the field of botany and its applications in medicine.

Background:

Medicinal Plant X, also known by its scientific name, Latinus plantus, has been used for centuries in traditional medicine to treat a wide range of ailments. Its unique chemical composition makes it a promising candidate for further investigation and potential use in modern medicine. Disease Y, on the other hand, affects millions of people worldwide, causing significant morbidity and mortality. Current treatment options for Disease Y are limited and often associated with undesirable side effects. Therefore, exploring alternative treatments, such as Medicinal Plant X, is crucial to finding more effective and safer therapeutic interventions.

Research   and   Findings:

Numerous studies have investigated the medicinal properties of Plant X in relation to Disease Y. The active compounds found in Plant X have shown promising results in various preclinical and clinical trials. For example, laboratory studies have demonstrated that specific compounds in Plant X possess anti-inflammatory properties, which could alleviate the symptoms associated with Disease Y. Additionally, other studies have indicated that Plant X extracts can inhibit the growth of certain pathogens linked to Disease Y, potentially offering a novel approach to combating the infection.

Practical   Applications: Understanding the potential of Plant X in treating Disease Y opens new avenues for student practitioners in botany. Research opportunities in this field include exploring the optimal extraction methods, investigating the mechanisms of action, and conducting further clinical trials to assess the safety and efficacy of Plant X-based treatments. This case study highlights the importance of bridging the gap between classroom knowledge and practical applications, empowering students to contribute to the development of novel therapies.

Conclusion:
In conclusion, Medicinal Plant X shows great promise in the treatment of Disease Y. As students in the field of botany, it is imperative that we continue to explore the potential of medicinal plants and their applications in modern medicine. By studying this case, we hope to inspire future practitioners to conduct further research, unravel the mysteries of these botanical wonders, and ultimately improve the lives of individuals affected by Disease Y. Remember, the classroom is just the beginning; the clinic awaits your contributions!

Case Study 2: Ethnobotanical Practices in a Specific Region

Introduction:
In the field of botany, the study of ethnobotanical practices provides valuable insights into how different cultures have utilized and benefited from medicinal plants throughout history. This case study will focus on a specific region and explore the fascinating relationship between people and plants, shedding light on traditional healing practices that have been passed down through generations.

Understanding   Ethnobotany:
Ethnobotany is the interdisciplinary study of the relationship between plants and people, emphasizing the knowledge and practices of indigenous communities regarding plant use for medicinal, cultural, and spiritual purposes. By examining ethnobotanical practices, we gain a deeper understanding of the importance of plant biodiversity and the ecological knowledge held by these communities.

Exploring   a   Specific   Region:
In this case study, we will delve into the ethnobotanical practices of the Amazon Rainforest, one of the world's most biodiverse regions. The indigenous tribes inhabiting this region have an intricate knowledge of the plants in their surroundings, utilizing them for a variety of medicinal purposes. We will explore their traditional healing practices, rituals, and the plants that play a crucial role in their daily lives.

Traditional   Medicinal   Plants:
The Amazon Rainforest is home to an extraordinary array of plant species with medicinal properties. We will discuss some of the most well-known plants used by indigenous tribes, such as the Cat's Claw

(Uncaria tomentosa) for its immune-boosting properties and Sangre de Grado (Croton lechleri) for wound healing. Understanding the therapeutic potential of these plants can pave the way for further research and the development of new pharmaceuticals.

Preserving   Traditional   Knowledge:
It is essential to recognize and respect the traditional knowledge of indigenous communities. By documenting and understanding their ethnobotanical practices, we can contribute to the preservation of their cultural heritage, while also benefiting from their valuable insights into plant medicine.

Conclusion:
Studying ethnobotanical practices in a specific region, such as the Amazon Rainforest, offers students of botany a unique opportunity to deepen their understanding of the relationship between humans and plants. By examining traditional healing practices and the utilization of medicinal plants, we can gain insights into the vast potential of botanical resources. Morcover, it is crucial to acknowledge and respect the traditional knowledge of indigenous communities, ensuring the preservation of their cultural heritage and the sustainable use of plant resources for future generations. This case study serves as a reminder of the interconnectedness between botany, cultural diversity, and the importance of protecting our planet's biodiversity.

Case Study 3: Integration of Medicinal Plants in Primary Healthcare

In recent years, there has been a growing interest in the integration of traditional medicinal plants into primary healthcare systems. This case study explores the potential benefits and challenges of incorporating medicinal plants into modern medical practices, specifically focusing on the field of botany.

As students of botany, it is crucial to understand the role that medicinal plants can play in improving healthcare outcomes. Traditional medicine has been used for centuries to treat various ailments, and many of these remedies are derived from plants. By studying the chemical properties and therapeutic effects of these plants, botanists can contribute valuable knowledge to the field of primary healthcare.

One example of successful integration is the use of Artemisia annua, commonly known as sweet wormwood, in the treatment of malaria. Traditional medicines derived from this plant have been used for centuries in certain parts of the world. However, it was only through the collaboration between botanists and medical practitioners that the active compound, artemisinin, was isolated and developed into a highly effective anti-malarial drug. This case study highlights the importance of interdisciplinary collaboration and the potential for botanical knowledge to contribute to medical advancements.

The integration of medicinal plants in primary healthcare also presents significant challenges. Standardization of plant-based remedies is essential to ensure consistent quality and efficacy. Botanists can play a crucial role in identifying the correct plant species, optimizing cultivation techniques, and developing quality control measures. Furthermore, there is a need for rigorous scientific research to validate the safety and efficacy of these botanical treatments, ensuring they meet the same standards as conventional pharmaceutical drugs.

For students of botany, this case study serves as a reminder of the responsibility we hold in bridging the gap between traditional plant-based medicines and modern healthcare. By embracing a holistic approach that combines traditional knowledge with scientific rigor, we can contribute to the development of evidence-based botanical therapies.

In conclusion, the integration of medicinal plants in primary healthcare offers immense potential for improving patient outcomes. As students of botany, we have a unique opportunity to contribute to this field by expanding our knowledge of medicinal plants, collaborating with medical practitioners, and conducting rigorous scientific research. By embracing this interdisciplinary approach, we can pave the way for a future where traditional and modern medicine coexist harmoniously, benefiting patients and the field of botany alike.

Chapter 9: Future Trends and Innovations in Medicinal Botany

Emerging Technologies in Medicinal Plant Research

In the ever-evolving field of medicinal botany, staying up-to-date with the latest advancements and technologies is crucial for students pursuing a career in this niche. With the rapid pace of scientific progress, emerging technologies have revolutionized the way we study and utilize medicinal plants. This subchapter aims to introduce students to some of the most significant technological advancements in medicinal plant research.

One of the most promising emerging technologies is genomics. The advent of next-generation sequencing techniques has enabled scientists to sequence the entire genome of medicinal plants, providing a wealth of genetic information. This technology helps identify important genes responsible for the production of bioactive compounds, allowing researchers to understand the biosynthetic pathways and potentially manipulate them for enhanced medicinal properties.

Another revolutionary technology is metabolomics, which involves the comprehensive analysis of the small molecules present in plants. By using cutting-edge mass spectrometry and nuclear magnetic resonance techniques, scientists can identify and quantify the diverse range of metabolites present in medicinal plants. This information is invaluable for characterizing the chemical composition of plant extracts, determining the presence of bioactive compounds, and understanding their role in human health.

Advancements in bioinformatics and computational biology have also greatly impacted medicinal plant research. These computational tools allow researchers to analyze large datasets, predict gene functions, and model metabolic pathways. By combining computational analyses with experimental validation, scientists can accelerate the discovery of potential medicinal compounds and optimize their production.

Furthermore, nanotechnology has emerged as a promising tool in medicinal plant research. Nanoparticles can be used to enhance the delivery of bioactive compounds, improve their solubility, and increase their stability. This technology has the potential to revolutionize drug delivery systems and treatment strategies by increasing the efficacy and bioavailability of medicinal plant-based drugs.

Lastly, the integration of artificial intelligence and machine learning algorithms has facilitated the identification of novel bioactive compounds from medicinal plants. These technologies can analyze vast databases of chemical structures and predict the potential therapeutic properties of compounds, thereby aiding in drug discovery and development.

In conclusion, the field of medicinal plant research is constantly evolving, and students interested in botany must stay abreast of the latest emerging technologies. Genomics, metabolomics, bioinformatics, nanotechnology, and artificial intelligence are just a few examples of game-changing technologies that are revolutionizing medicinal botany. By understanding and utilizing these tools, students can contribute to the discovery and development of novel drugs derived from medicinal plants, ultimately improving human health and well-being.

Biotechnological Approaches in Medicinal Botany

In recent years, the field of medicinal botany has witnessed significant advancements with the integration of biotechnological approaches. These approaches have revolutionized the way we study and utilize medicinal plants, offering immense potential for drug discovery and development. As students of botany, it is crucial to understand the role of biotechnology in this field and its implications for future research and practice.

One of the most promising biotechnological approaches in medicinal botany is plant tissue culture. This technique involves the aseptic culture of plant cells, tissues, or organs in a controlled environment. It enables the production of large quantities of uniform and disease-free plant material, which can serve as a renewable source for valuable secondary metabolites, such as alkaloids, flavonoids, and terpenoids. Tissue culture also allows for the genetic manipulation of plants, leading to the enhancement of desired traits and the production of novel compounds with therapeutic potential.

Another biotechnological tool that has revolutionized medicinal botany is genetic engineering. By introducing foreign genes into plants, researchers can enhance their medicinal properties or introduce entirely new biosynthetic pathways. This technique has been successfully employed to boost the production of bioactive compounds, such as artemisinin in Artemisia annua, a plant used in the treatment of malaria. Genetic engineering also holds promise for the development of plants with enhanced tolerance to environmental stresses, thus ensuring a more sustainable and reliable supply of medicinal plants.

Furthermore, biotechnological approaches have paved the way for the establishment of plant molecular farming. This innovative concept involves the production of pharmaceuticals, vaccines, and other therapeutic proteins using genetically modified plants as bioreactors. By harnessing the plant's natural ability to produce complex molecules, this approach offers a cost-effective and scalable alternative to traditional manufacturing methods. Plant molecular farming holds great potential for addressing global health challenges, particularly in developing countries where access to essential medicines is limited.

As students passionate about botany, embracing biotechnological approaches in medicinal plant research is essential. These approaches not only offer exciting research opportunities but also have the potential to make a significant impact on human health. By combining our knowledge of plant biology with biotechnological tools, we can unlock the full potential of medicinal plants and contribute to the development of safer and more effective drugs. As future practitioners, let us embrace these advancements and strive to bridge the gap between classroom learning and clinical applications, ultimately making a positive difference in the field of medicinal botany.

Potential Applications of Medicinal Botany in Personalized Medicine

In recent years, personalized medicine has emerged as a promising approach to healthcare, aiming to provide tailored treatments based on an individual's unique genetic makeup, lifestyle, and environment. Within this field, medicinal botany plays a crucial role in the identification, extraction, and utilization of plant-based compounds for personalized therapeutic interventions. This subchapter explores the potential applications of medicinal botany in personalized medicine, shedding light on the ways in which students in the field of botany can contribute to this exciting and rapidly evolving field.

One of the key areas where medicinal botany is making significant contributions to personalized medicine is in the discovery and development of novel drugs. Plants have a rich history of being a source of various bioactive compounds, many of which possess therapeutic properties. By studying plant biodiversity and employing advanced techniques such as high-throughput screening and bioassays, botany students can identify and characterize new medicinal compounds. These compounds can then be further studied for their potential in personalized medicine, allowing for targeted treatments based on an individual's specific molecular profile.

Moreover, medicinal botany also plays a crucial role in understanding the mechanisms of action of plant-derived compounds. By investigating how these compounds interact with biological systems, botany students can contribute to the development of personalized medicine approaches that optimize drug effectiveness while minimizing adverse effects. This knowledge can further aid in the development of personalized treatment plans, ensuring that patients receive the most suitable interventions based on their genetic predispositions and other individual factors.

In addition to drug discovery and mechanism studies, medicinal botany can also contribute to personalized medicine through the identification of botanical markers for disease risk and prognosis. By studying the relationship between specific plant compounds and certain health conditions, botany students can help identify biomarkers that can be used for early disease detection and personalized risk assessment. This information can then be integrated into diagnostic tools and treatment algorithms, allowing for more accurate and personalized healthcare interventions.

Overall, the potential applications of medicinal botany in personalized medicine are vast. From drug discovery to understanding mechanisms of action and identifying biomarkers, students in the field of botany have a unique opportunity to contribute to this exciting and rapidly advancing field. By harnessing the power of plants and their bioactive compounds, personalized medicine can revolutionize healthcare by providing tailored treatments that improve patient outcomes and minimize adverse effects. As future practitioners, botany students have a critical role to play in shaping the future of personalized medicine, making this an exciting and promising area of study and practice.

Chapter 10: Conclusion and Practical Applications

Recapitulation of Key Concepts

As we near the end of our journey through the world of medicinal botany, it is essential to recapitulate the key concepts we have explored. This subchapter aims to provide students with a comprehensive overview of the fundamental principles and practices covered in this book, "From Classroom to Clinic: Medicinal Botany for Student Practitioners."

Botany, the scientific study of plants, plays a pivotal role in understanding the medicinal properties and potential of various plant species. Throughout this book, we have delved into the intricate relationship between medicinal plants and human health. By examining the chemical compounds present in plants, their therapeutic properties, and the methods of their extraction, we have gained valuable insights into the field of medicinal botany.

In our exploration, we have learned about the classification and identification of medicinal plants, including their taxonomy and nomenclature. Understanding how to identify different plant families and species is crucial for accurate botanical research and the development of effective herbal medicines. We have also discussed the importance of plant conservation and sustainable harvesting practices to ensure the longevity of these valuable resources.

Furthermore, we have delved into the chemical constituents present in medicinal plants and their potential therapeutic applications. From alkaloids to flavonoids, terpenoids to phenolics, we have explored the diverse range of compounds that contribute to the healing properties of plants. Students have gained a deeper understanding of how these compounds interact with the human body, including their mechanism of action and potential side effects.

In addition to plant identification and chemical constituents, we have covered various extraction methods used in medicinal botany. From traditional techniques such as maceration and decoction to modern advancements like supercritical fluid extraction and chromatography, students have learned about the different approaches to obtain plant extracts rich in bioactive compounds.

To ensure the safety and efficacy of medicinal plant products, we have emphasized the importance of quality control and standardization. This includes the evaluation of plant material, extraction processes, and the implementation of Good Manufacturing Practices (GMP) to guarantee consistent and reliable herbal medicines.

In conclusion, this subchapter on the recapitulation of key concepts serves as a comprehensive review for students studying medicinal botany. By revisiting the fundamental principles and practices covered in this book, students can reinforce their understanding of important topics such as plant identification, chemical constituents, extraction methods, and quality control. Armed with this knowledge, future student practitioners will be well-equipped to navigate the fascinating world of medicinal botany and contribute to the advancement of herbal medicine.

Recommendations for Student Practitioners

As a student of botany, you are embarking on an exciting journey into the world of medicinal plants. The field of medicinal botany offers a unique opportunity to combine your passion for plants with the practical application of herbal remedies. To help you make the most of this experience, here are some recommendations for student practitioners like yourself.

1. Develop a strong foundation in botany: Before diving into the world of medicinal botany, it is essential to have a solid understanding of basic botany principles. Familiarize yourself with plant anatomy, taxonomy, and physiology. This knowledge will serve as a strong foundation for your future studies and practice.

2. Study local flora: Gain a comprehensive understanding of the botanical diversity in your region. Identify and study the medicinal plants native to your area. This will allow you to develop a deeper connection with the local ecosystem and its healing potential.

3. Learn from experienced practitioners: Seek out mentors or experienced practitioners in the field of medicinal botany. Their guidance and expertise can provide invaluable insights and help you avoid common pitfalls. Attend workshops, conferences, and seminars to network with professionals and learn from their experiences.

4. Hands-on experience: Actively engage in fieldwork and practical exercises. Visit botanical gardens, nature reserves, and herbal farms to observe and learn about medicinal plants in their natural habitats. Cultivate your own medicinal garden to gain firsthand experience in growing and caring for medicinal plants.

5. Ethical considerations: Ethical harvesting and sustainable practices are crucial in the field of medicinal botany. Respect the plants and their habitats by practicing responsible harvesting techniques and promoting sustainability. Learn about the conservation efforts in place and contribute to the preservation of medicinal plant species.

6. Keep a journal: Maintain a detailed journal of your experiences, observations, and findings. Document the properties, uses, and preparations of different medicinal plants. This will serve as a valuable resource for future reference and help you track your progress as a student practitioner.

7. Continual learning: Stay updated with the latest research and developments in the field of medicinal botany. Subscribe to relevant journals, join professional organizations, and participate in online forums or discussion groups. Continually expand your knowledge and skills to stay at the forefront of this ever-evolving field.

Remember, as a student practitioner, you have the potential to make a significant impact on the field of medicinal botany. Embrace these recommendations and immerse yourself fully in the world of botanical medicine. Your dedication and passion will pave the way for a rewarding and fulfilling career in medicinal botany.

Prospect for Further Research in Medicinal Botany

As students pursuing a career in botany, it is essential to explore the prospect of further research in the field of medicinal botany. Medicinal botany is a fascinating area that combines the study of plants with their potential therapeutic properties. With the increasing demand for natural and sustainable healthcare alternatives, the significance of medicinal botany has never been more crucial.

One exciting prospect for further research in medicinal botany is the exploration of traditional plant-based remedies. Many traditional healing practices, such as Ayurveda and Traditional Chinese Medicine, have utilized plants for centuries to treat various ailments. By studying these traditional remedies and their active compounds, we can gain valuable insights into the potential therapeutic applications of plants. This research could lead to the identification of new compounds and the development of novel drugs.

Furthermore, the discovery of new plant species and their potential medicinal properties presents an exciting avenue for research. With vast areas of our planet unexplored, there is a high likelihood of discovering previously unknown plant species that may hold significant medicinal value. Exploring these uncharted territories and studying the chemical composition of these plants can provide us with a plethora of new therapeutic possibilities.

In addition to discovering new plant species, advancements in technology have opened up new avenues for research in medicinal botany. Techniques such as metabolomics and genomics allow us to study the chemical composition and genetic makeup of plants in a more detailed and efficient manner. By applying these cutting-edge technologies, we can uncover the intricate relationships between plant compounds and their potential medicinal effects.

Moreover, the field of medicinal botany also offers opportunities for interdisciplinary research. Collaborations with other scientific disciplines such as pharmacology, biochemistry, and ethnobotany can provide a holistic approach to understanding the therapeutic potential of plants. By combining the expertise of various fields, we can accelerate the discovery and development of new drugs derived from plants.

In conclusion, the prospect for further research in medicinal botany is vast and promising. As students in the field of botany, we have the opportunity to delve into traditional plant-based remedies, explore uncharted territories, utilize advanced technologies, and engage in interdisciplinary research. By embracing these prospects, we can contribute to the ever-growing field of medicinal botany and pave the way for the development of effective and sustainable healthcare solutions.

www.ingramcontent.com/pod-product-compliance
Lightning Source LLC
Chambersburg PA
CBHW051353150726
48000CB00003B/1160